Acne Keloidalis Nuchae

A Beginner's 3-Step Quick Start Plan to Managing AKN Through Diet, With Sample Recipes and a 7-Day Meal Plan

mf

copyright © 2022 Jeffrey Winzant

All rights reserved No part of this book may be reproduced, or stored in a retrieval system, or transmitted in any form or by any means, electronic, mechanical, photocopying, recording, or otherwise, without express written permission of the publisher.

Disclaimer

By reading this disclaimer, you are accepting the terms of the disclaimer in full. If you disagree with this disclaimer, please do not read the guide.

All of the content within this guide is provided for informational and educational purposes only, and should not be accepted as independent medical or other professional advice. The author is not a doctor, physician, nurse, mental health provider, or registered nutritionist/dietician. Therefore, using and reading this guide does not establish any form of a physician-patient relationship.

Always consult with a physician or another qualified health provider with any issues or questions you might have regarding any sort of medical condition. Do not ever disregard any qualified professional medical advice or delay seeking that advice because of anything you have read in this guide. The information in this guide is not intended to be any sort of medical advice and should not be used in lieu of any medical advice by a licensed and qualified medical professional.

The information in this guide has been compiled from a variety of known sources. However, the author cannot attest to or guarantee the accuracy of each source and thus should not be held liable for any errors or omissions.

You acknowledge that the publisher of this guide will not be held liable for any loss or damage of any kind incurred as a result of this guide or the reliance on any information provided within this guide. You acknowledge and agree that you assume all risk and responsibility for any action you undertake in response to the information in this guide.

Using this guide does not guarantee any particular result (e.g., weight loss or a cure). By reading this guide, you acknowledge that there are no guarantees to any specific outcome or results you can expect.

All product names, diet plans, or names used in this guide are for identification purposes only and are the property of their respective owners. The use of these names does not imply endorsement. All other trademarks cited herein are the property of their respective owners.

Where applicable, this guide is not intended to be a substitute for the original work of this diet plan and is, at most, a supplement to the original work for this diet plan and never a direct substitute. This guide is a personal expression of the facts of that diet plan.

Where applicable, persons shown in the cover images are stock photography models and the publisher has obtained the rights to use the images through license agreements with third-party stock image companies.

Table of Contents

Introduction	6
All About Acne Keloidalis Nuchae	8
Diagnosis and Treatments	11
Medical Treatments	11
Ways to Manage AKN	13
3-Step Plan for Managing AKN	13
Eating a Healthy Diet	14
7-Day Meal Plan	18
Use of Natural Treatments	19
Lifestyle Changes	21
Sample Recipes	26
Tuna and Veggies Wrap	27
Grenade Salad	28
Spinach, Feta, and Tomato Omelet	29
Vegetarian Casserole	30
Sun Crust Turkey Cuts	32
No-Fuss Tuna Casserole	34
Baked Flounder	35
Tangy Lemon Fish	36
Horseradish Aioli and Roast Beef Sandwich	38
Kale Fried Rice	39
Stir-Fried Cabbage and Apples	41
Roast Broccoli and Salmon	42
Asian-Themed Macrobiotic Bowl	44
Spinach Quiche	46
Grilled Eggplant	48
Conclusion	49
FAQ About Acne Keloidalis Nuchae	50
References and Helpful Links	52

Introduction

Acne keloidalis nuchae, also known as AKN, is a condition that leads to the development of bumps on the back of the neck that resemble keloids. These bumps can be both painful and itchy, and they have the potential to occasionally get in the way of day-to-day activities. AKN is most prevalent in people of African descent; however, it is not exclusive to those people of African descent and can occur in people of other ethnicities as well.

There is currently no treatment that can reverse the effects of AKN, but there are ways to manage the condition and slow down its symptoms. The management of AKN relies heavily on maintaining a healthy diet and lifestyle. In addition, several natural treatments can help to lessen the bumps and improve the skin's overall appearance.

In this quick start guide, we will discuss AKN in detail. We will also provide a 3-step plan for managing AKN through diet and other natural lifestyle changes.

In this guide, you will discover:

- What causes acne keloidalis nuchae (AKN)
- What are its symptoms
- How AKN is diagnosed
- What are the treatments for AKN
- How can it be prevented
- The 3-step plan on how to manage acne keloidalis nuchae through diet, natural treatments, and lifestyle changes

All About Acne Keloidalis Nuchae

It is believed that AKN is brought on by a combination of factors, the most significant of which are genetic factors, inflammation, and damage to the hair follicles. Understanding these risk factors is essential for the development of effective treatments for AKN, even though the precise cause of AKN is not yet known.

- *Genetic Predisposition:* The exact cause of AKN is unknown, but it is believed to be associated with a combination of genetic and environmental factors. People of African descent are more likely to develop AKN due to their genetic predisposition. This is because people of African descent tend to have higher levels of certain inflammatory chemicals in their skin. In addition, AKN is more common in people who have a history of acne or other skin conditions.
- *Inflammation:* AKN is thought to be related to chronic inflammation of the hair follicles. When the body gets hurt or sick, its natural response is inflammation. It can make your skin red, swell up, and hurt.

The inflammatory response is a complicated process that involves immune cells becoming active and inflammatory mediators being released. Even though inflammation is necessary and can be helpful, too much of it can damage tissues and cause disease. Because of this, it's important to know how inflammation happens and how to stop it.

- ***Trauma to the Hair Follicles:*** Keloids are a type of tumor that develops when the body produces an abnormally high amount of collagen in response to an injury. It is believed that AKN is brought on by repetitive trauma to the hair follicles, such as that caused by wearing one's hair in a ponytail or by shaving. The follicles are harmed as a result of this trauma, which also makes them more susceptible to infection. Keloids are sometimes formed as a consequence of the inflammation that this condition causes.

Although the cause of AKN is unknown, it is thought to be caused by a combination of these factors. If you are experiencing this condition, it is important to seek medical attention from a dermatologist who can help you develop a treatment plan.

Symptoms

The main symptom of AKN is the formation of keloid-like bumps on the back of the neck. These bumps can range in size from a few millimeters to several centimeters. They may be flesh-colored, pink, red, or brown. The bumps can be itchy and painful, and they may bleed if scratched.

AKN can also cause hair loss on the back of the neck. This is because the keloid-like bumps can damage the hair follicles. In severe cases, AKN can lead to scarring and disfigurement of the back of the neck.

Diagnosis and Treatments

Acne keloidalis nuchae is a condition that causes scarring and inflammation on the back of the neck and the scalp. No one test can definitively diagnose the condition, but a medical professional can typically determine it after considering the patient's symptoms and performing a physical exam.

The healthcare provider will inquire as to when the symptoms first appeared, whether or not they have evolved, what causes the skin to become irritated, as well as the treatments that have already been attempted. If the diagnosis is unclear, the healthcare provider may suggest further testing, such as a biopsy or culture, to assist in confirming the diagnosis.

Medical Treatments

Although AKN has no known cure, the condition is typically managed with medications that reduce symptoms. Here are some of the medical treatments that can be used to manage AKN:

- ***Antibiotics:*** Antibiotics, either topically applied or taken orally, may be used to treat or prevent bacterial infection.
- ***Retinoids:*** Retinoids may be used to improve overall symptoms. Retinoids are a class of drugs that are derived from vitamin A. They work by reducing inflammation and regulating cell turnover. In addition, retinoids can help to reduce the appearance of scars.
- ***Steroids:*** Steroids help to reduce inflammation and can be taken orally or injected directly into the affected area.
- ***Surgical excision:*** If the condition does not respond to medical treatment, surgical options may be considered. This may involve the removal of scar tissue, as well as the administration of injections to break up the fibrous bands that can cause the scars to form.

Other potential treatments, such as radiotherapy, laser therapy, phototherapy, and laser hair removal, are also being investigated and tested by researchers.

With proper treatment, acne keloidalis nuchae can be effectively managed. However, recurrence is possible, so long-term care is often necessary to keep the condition under control.

Ways to Manage AKN

There is no full-proof way to avoid getting AKN, but there are some things you can do to decrease the chances of getting it. If you are of African descent, you should steer clear of hairstyles that pull your hair back too tightly and avoid shaving your head. In addition, you should make an effort to reduce the amount of inflammation present in your skin by eating a healthy diet and making use of gentle skincare products.

3-Step Plan for Managing AKN

If you are experiencing AKN, there are a few things you can do to manage the condition and reduce the symptoms. Here is a 3-step plan for managing AKN:

1. Eat a healthy diet

Eating a healthy diet is important for managing AKN. Foods that are rich in antioxidants, such as fruits and vegetables, can help to reduce inflammation. In addition, you should try to avoid processed foods and foods that are high in sugar.

2. Use natural treatments

Several natural treatments can help to reduce the bumps and improve the appearance of the skin. These treatments include aloe vera, tea tree oil, and vitamin E.

3. Lifestyle Changes

In addition to diet and natural treatments, there are a few lifestyle changes you can make to help manage AKN. These changes include avoiding tight hairstyles and shaving and limiting the amount of inflammation in your skin.

By following these steps, you can help to reduce the symptoms of AKN and improve the appearance of your skin.

Eating a Healthy Diet

A healthy diet is important for managing AKN. Eating a diet that is high in fresh fruits and vegetables, lean protein, and healthy fats can help to reduce inflammation and improve the appearance of the skin. In addition, avoiding processed foods, sugary drinks, and excessive alcohol consumption is important for managing AKN.

Foods to Eat

- ***Fresh fruits*** are high in antioxidants and vitamins that can help to reduce inflammation. Antioxidants scavenge harmful byproducts of cellular metabolism known as free radicals, which can damage cells, leading to inflammation.

Vitamins A, C, and E are particularly effective at reducing inflammation. Vitamin C is found in abundance in citrus fruits such as oranges and grapefruit.

Vitamin E is found in nuts and seeds, while carrots and sweet potatoes are good sources of vitamin A.

In addition to these nutrients, fresh fruits also contain fiber, which can help to regulate digestion and reduce inflammation throughout the body. When it comes to fighting inflammation, fresh fruits are nature's superheroes.

- *Vegetables:* Vegetables are a powerhouse when it comes to skincare. They are a good source of fiber, which can help to improve the appearance of the skin. In addition, vegetables are high in vitamins and minerals that can help to reduce inflammation. For example, beta-carotene, which is found in carrots, sweet potatoes, and kale, can help to protect the skin from sun damage. Similarly, vitamin C, which is found in peppers, broccoli, and spinach, can help to brighten the skin.

- *Lean protein:* When it comes to a healthy diet, lean protein is an essential component. Not only does it help to reduce inflammation, but it can also improve the appearance of the skin. In addition, lean protein helps to promote a healthy weight by boosting metabolism and preventing cravings. While there are many sources of lean protein, some of the best include fish,chicken, and beans.

When selecting lean protein, it is important to choose quality over quantity. Look for a protein that is free of hormones and antibiotics, and be sure to cook it healthily.

- *Healthy fats:* Inflammation is a process by which the body's white blood cells and chemicals protect us from infection and foreign substances. However, when inflammation occurs in the body on a chronic basis, it can lead to several health problems, such as heart disease and arthritis.

One way to help reduce inflammation is to consume healthy fats, such as omega-3 fatty acids. Olive oil, avocados, nuts, and seeds are also good options. These essential nutrients help to regulate the inflammatory response and can also have several other benefits, such as improving the appearance of the skin.

In addition, healthy fats are an important part of a balanced diet and can help to promote overall health.

Foods to Avoid

- *Processed foods:* Processed foods are those that have been altered from their natural state in some way, such as by canning, freezing, or adding preservatives. Though they may be convenient, these foods are often high in sugar and unhealthy fats that can trigger inflammation.

  Inflammation is a response by the body's immune system to protect against infection or injury. However, when it becomes chronic, it can lead to several health problems. For these reasons, it's best to limit processed foods in your diet and focus on eating fresh, whole foods instead.

- *Sugary drinks:* When you have AKN, it is important to be extra careful about what you eat and drink. Sugary drinks, such as soda and fruit juice, are high in sugar and calories. They can also trigger inflammation. This can make your AKN worse. It is best to avoid sugary drinks altogether, or at least limit them to small occasional servings.

- *Excessive alcohol consumption:* Consuming alcohol in large quantities regularly may make your AKN symptoms even more severe. Because alcohol is a diuretic, it causes the body to expel water through the urinary tract. If you don't drink enough water, your body will start to dehydrate, which will cause your skin to become dry and flaky, making it more prone to irritation and infection.

In addition, drinking alcohol can lead to changes in hormone levels, which can also cause acne keloidalis nuchae or make existing cases of the condition worse.

7-Day Meal Plan

Below is a sample 7-day meal plan that you can either follow or modify, depending on your preference. Take note that you don't have to strictly prepare one recipe per meal. You can save leftovers and eat them for later.

Meal	Breakfast	Lunch	Dinner
Day 1	Spinach Quiche	Tuna and Veggies Wrap	Roast Broccoli and Salmon
Day 2	Horseradish Aioli and Roast Beef Sandwich	Asian-Themed Macrobiotic Bowl	Tangy Lemon Fish
Day 3	Spinach, Feta, and Tomato Omelet	Stir-Fried Cabbage and Apples	Sun Crust Turkey Cuts
Day 4	Vegetarian Casserole	Kale Fried Rice	Spinach, Feta, and Tomato Omelet
Day 5	Grilled Eggplant	Spinach Quiche	Baked Flounder

| Day 6 | Grenade Salad | No-Fuss Tuna Casserole | Asian-Themed Macrobiotic Bowl |
| Day 7 | Tuna and Veggies Wrap | Horseradish Aioli and Roast Beef Sandwich | Kale Fried Rice |

Use of Natural Treatments

Several natural treatments can help to reduce the bumps and improve the appearance of the skin. These treatments include:

- *Tea tree oil:* Tea tree oil has natural properties that make it effective as both an antiseptic and an anti-inflammatory agent. It can be put on the bumps topically to help reduce swelling and redness in those areas. Tea tree oil can be used by the vast majority of people without risk when it is applied in the recommended manner.

    On the other hand, this medication may cause skin irritation or other adverse effects in some people. Before using tea tree oil, you should discuss your concerns about any potential adverse reactions with your attending physician or pharmacist.

- *Aloe vera:* Aloe vera is a type of succulent that grows perennially and has been cultivated for its medicinal qualities for hundreds of years. Burns, inflammation, and insect bites are all conditions that can be relieved by topically applying the gel that is extracted from the plant's leaves. In addition to that, it can be taken in the form of juice or gel to assist with digestive problems.

Because it contains a high concentration of vitamins, minerals, and antioxidants, aloe vera is a potent natural remedy for a variety of conditions. It is not difficult to cultivate your aloe vera plant, despite the fact that this plant is found in a wide variety of over-the-counter products. Aloe vera is a plant that requires little in the way of care and tending and does best in hot, sunny climates. You can treat your own AKN symptoms, such as inflammation, naturally at home with just a little bit of effort and attention to detail.

- *Apple cider vinegar:* Apple cider vinegar is a natural remedy that has properties that make it effective against both bacteria and inflammation. It is possible to dilute it with water and then apply it topically to the bumps in order to assist in reducing the redness and swelling. Acetic acid, which is found in apple cider vinegar, has been shown to be effective in reducing inflammation and killing bacteria. In addition to that, it has malic acid, which can aid in the exfoliation of the skin and the opening of clogged pores.

- *Coconut oil:* Coconut oil is a natural moisturizer that can be utilized to help in keeping the skin hydrated.

The bumps can be treated topically with it, or it can be taken orally in very small doses. Coconut oil is full of nourishing fatty acids that are great for protecting and nourishing the skin. These acids not only help to prevent dryness but also help to provide moisture.

Additionally, because it has anti-inflammatory properties, coconut oil can help reduce redness and swelling in the affected area. Coconut oil, when used topically, can calm the skin and diminish the appearance of bumps. It has been shown that consuming it in moderate amounts can help improve the skin's overall health.

Lifestyle Changes

In addition to a healthy diet and natural treatments, several lifestyle changes can help to reduce the symptoms of AKN. These lifestyle changes include:

- *Avoiding tight hairstyles:* A condition known as acne keloidalis nuchae (AKN) is characterized by the development of scar tissue around the hair follicles as a result of the condition. If treatment is not pursued the condition can result in irreversible balding in men of African descent, who are more likely to be affected by it. It is not known for certain what causes AKN; however, researchers believe that it is brought on by excessive stress placed on the hair follicles over time.

One of the most common causes of AKN is the use of tight hairstyles, which can cause damage to the hair follicles and make the symptoms of the condition worse. Therefore, people who have AKN should steer clear of having their hair pulled back into tight ponytails, braids, or cornrows.

Those who are at risk of developing AKN should also take extra precautions to prevent their scalps from being injured through repeated trauma. When venturing outside, it is a good idea to protect yourself from the sun by donning a hat or scarf.

- *Avoiding shaving:* The symptoms of AKN are often something that patients with the condition have to cope with daily. The appearance of bumps on the skin is both one of the most evident and one of the most bothersome symptoms. These lumps can cause a great deal of discomfort, and they may make it difficult for those who have them to go about their normal daily activities.

  In certain instances, razor burn can also make the symptoms of AKN significantly worse. Because of this, it is essential to proceed with caution whenever one shaves. If at all possible, you should refrain from shaving over the bumps. If you absolutely must shave, make sure your razor is sharp and steer clear of the bumps on your skin. This will not only help to keep the symptoms of AKN under control, but it will also help to reduce the likelihood of getting razor burn.

- ***Wearing loose clothing:*** Acne keloidalis nuchae, also known as AKN, is a condition that manifests itself as raised bumps on the nape of the neck. The bumps almost always itch and can sometimes be quite uncomfortable. The bumps may become infected, which will then result in scarring.

   Wearing clothing that is too tight can make the symptoms of AKN worse because it irritates the bumps and makes the condition worse overall. It is essential to dress in loose-fitting clothing, such as shirts made of cotton, as this is the most comfortable option. Wearing clothing that is loose and comfortable is one way to help keep the bumps clean and dry while also contributing to a reduction in irritation.

   Additionally, it is essential to avoid sharing hats, towels, or any other personal items with someone who has AKN because doing so can spread the infection. Sharing can cause the virus to become more widespread. By practicing the appropriate precautions, not only will you be able to protect the health of your own skin, but you will also be helping the fight against the further spread of AKN.

- *Avoiding hot showers:* Spending a long, hot shower might feel relaxing, but it can be bad for your skin. Hot water can strip away the natural oils that protect your skin, leading to dryness, irritation, and even dermatitis. And if you have acne-prone skin, hot showers can make your condition worse by causing the sebaceous glands to produce more oil.

  To keep your skin healthy, it's best to stick to lukewarm showers and avoid scrubbing too vigorously. When you do wash, focus on areas that tend to be oily or sweaty, such as the face, chest, and back. And be sure to moisturize afterward to help lock in hydration. By following these simple tips, you can keep your skin looking and feeling its best.

- *Avoiding sunlight:* It might be soothing to take a long, hot shower, but doing so frequently can be damaging to your skin. The natural oils that protect your skin from damage can be removed by washing with hot water, which can result in dryness, irritation, and even dermatitis. In addition, if you have acne-prone skin, taking hot showers can make your condition even more severe because they trigger the sebaceous glands to produce more oil.

  Showering in lukewarm water and avoiding vigorous exfoliation are two of the most effective ways to preserve the health of your skin. When you do wash, pay particular attention to areas of the face, chest, and back that have a propensity for producing oil or sweat. And don't forget to apply a moisturizer afterward to help seal in the moisture. You can maintain the healthiest looking and feeling skin possible by adhering to these few easy guidelines.

Altering certain aspects of one's lifestyle can also be beneficial in the fight against AKN and its symptoms. These lifestyle changes include staying away from hairstyles that are too constricting, shaving, wearing loose clothing, and taking cooler showers. Discuss the various treatment options with your physician if you are having trouble keeping your AKN under control.

Sample Recipes

Tuna and Veggies Wrap

Ingredients:

- 1 canned tuna
- 2 pcs. whole-grain tortillas
- 1 cup cucumber, sliced
- 1 tbsp. low-fat Italian dressing
- 1 cup carrots, julienned

Instructions:

1. Put the dressing and tuna in a bowl and mix well.
2. Arrange half of the mixture on one of the tortillas. Add half the amount of each vegetable and wrap.
3. Do the same to the remaining tortilla.

Grenade Salad

Ingredients:

- 4 cups arugula
- 1 large avocado
- 1/2 cup sliced fennel
- 1/2 cup sliced Anjou pears
- /4 cup pomegranate seeds

Instructions:

1. Mix all the ingredients except for the pomegranate seeds.
2. After mixing well, add the seeds. Mix again.
3. Serve with any type of desired dressing.

Spinach, Feta, and Tomato Omelet

Ingredients:

- cooking spray
- 1/4 cup Roma tomatoes, chopped
- 3/4 cup Egg Beaters Liquid Egg Whites
- 2 tbsp. fat reduced feta cheese, crumbled
- 1/8 tsp. ground black pepper
- 1/4 cup baby spinach leaves, chopped

Instructions:

1. Spray small amounts of cooking spray in a nonstick skillet. Heat over medium heat.
2. Cook the Egg Beaters in the skillet, season with pepper. Cook for 2 minutes.
3. Lift the edges to cook the other side of the egg. Cook for 3 more minutes.
4. Top the half of the omelet with tomatoes, spinach, and feta cheese. Fold the other half of the omelet over the filling.
5. Serve.

Vegetarian Casserole

Ingredients:

- 1 medium-sized sweet potato
- 1/2 small cauliflower head
- 1/2 tsp. cumin seeds
- 1 small onion
- 1 red bell pepper
- 1 tbsp. olive oil or extra virgin olive oil
- 1-1/4 cup of red salsa
- 5 corn tortillas
- 1/2 can black beans
- 1/4 cup chopped cilantro
- 1 handful of spinach leaves
- 1/2 cup of Shredded Monterey Jack

Instructions:

1. Oven-roast vegetables at 400°F. Place the vegetables on a baking sheet to avoid sticking.
2. Mix cauliflower head together with cut sweet potato and olive oil in a pan.
3. Heat another pan and mix bell pepper, onion, and olive oil on it. Add cumin seeds to both pans.
4. Drizzle salt and pepper to taste in both pans. Ensure that the mixture becomes coated in spices.

5. Add olive oil whenever you think it is necessary. Oven-bake until vegetables are tender and caramelized.
6. Mix the cilantro with the red salsa. Lower oven temperature to 350°F.
7. Pour in the salsa onto the bottom of the pan. Place a layer of tortilla and make sure it is covered with salsa.
8. Add in the beans, vegetables, spinach and cheese.
9. Carefully create another tortilla layer and pour in all of the remaining salsa, vegetables, and Monterey Jack.
10. Repeat the process and cover the pan with parchment paper.
11. Bake for 20 minutes and remove the cover.
12. After a few minutes of cooling down, return the pan back into the oven and heat for another 10 minutes.
13. Remove the pan from the oven and let the casserole cool and dry before serving.

Sun Crust Turkey Cuts

Ingredients:

- 2 turkey breasts, cut into 1/4-inch thick slices
- 1-1/2 cups sunflower seeds
- 1/4 tsp. ground cumin
- 2 tbsp. chopped parsley
- 1/4 tsp. paprika
- 1/4 tsp. cayenne pepper
- 1/4 tsp. black pepper
- 1/3 cup whole wheat flour
- 3 egg whites

Instructions:

1. Preheat the oven to around 395 °F.
2. Mix the parsley, paprika, cumin, cayenne, sunflower seeds, and pepper in a processor.
3. Prepare the whites and flour in a separate container each.
4. Coat each breast part with the mixtures separately. Start with the flour mixture, followed by the whites, and then the processed mixture.
5. After coating all the breasts, prepare the pan.

6. Bake the breasts for approximately 12 minutes in the oven.
7. Flip each side and resume baking for another 12 minutes.
8. Serve hot.

No-Fuss Tuna Casserole

Ingredients:

- 1-5 oz. can tuna, drained
- 1 can cream of chicken soup, condensed
- 3 cups macaroni, cooked
- 1-1/2 cups fried onions
- 1 cup Cheddar cheese, shredded

Instructions:

1. Preheat the oven to 350°F.
2. Prepare a 9x13-inch baking dish. Use that to mix the macaroni, tuna, and soup. Top it with cheese.
3. Bake for 25 minutes or until the casserole is bubbly.
4. Sprinkle it with fried onions. Put back in the oven and leave for 5 more minutes.
5. Serve and enjoy while hot.

Baked Flounder

Ingredients:

- 1 lb. flounder, fileted
- 1/4 tsp. salt
- 1 cup halved red grapes
- 1 tbsp. extra-virgin olive oil
- 2 tbsp. parsley, chopped finely
- 1 tbsp. lemon juice
- 1 cup almonds, chopped and toasted
- freshly ground black pepper, to taste

Instructions:

1. Preheat the oven to 375°F.
2. Place fish on a sheet tray. Season with olive oil, salt, and pepper.
3. Combine the almonds, grapes, lemon juice, parsley, 1-1/2 tsp. of olive oil, 1/8 tsp of salt, and black pepper in a bowl.
4. Bake the fish for about 3 minutes.
5. Flip the fish and return it to the oven.
6. Bake for another 3 minutes, or until the fish is starting to flake, while the center is still translucent. Don't overcook.
7. Serve immediately, topped with the grape mixture.

Tangy Lemon Fish

Ingredients:

- 200 g. Gurnard fresh fish filets
- 3 tbsp. butter
- 1 tbsp. fresh lemon juice
- 1/4 cup fine almond flour
- 1 tsp. dried dill
- 1 tsp. dried chives
- 1 tsp. onion powder
- 1/2 tsp. garlic powder
- salt
- pepper

Instructions:

1. On a large plate or tray, combine dill, almond flour, and spices. Mix until well combined.
2. Dredge each file one at a time into the flour mix. Turn the filet around until fully coated, and then transfer it to a clean plate or tray. This may be refrigerated until ready to cook.
3. Place a large pan over medium-high heat.
4. Combine halves of butter and lemon juice. Swirl the pan to mix, and lift occasionally to avoid burning the butter.
5. Allow the fish to cook for about 3 minutes.

6. Let the fish absorb all the lemony-butter mixture. Cook on low heat to avoid drying out the pan.
7. Add the remaining lemon juice and butter to the pan.
8. Turn the fish to cook the other side for 3 minutes more. Swirl around the pan to fully coat it with the juice.
9. Wait until it turns golden brown and the fish is cooked through.
10. Serve with buttered vegetables.

Horseradish Aioli and Roast Beef Sandwich

Ingredients:

- 1 tbsp. low-fat, less sodium Italian dressing
- 2 oz. roast beef, sliced
- 2 tbsp. reduced-fat mayonnaise
- 1 small cucumber, sliced
- 2 slices rye bread
- 1/2 cup fresh spinach
- 2 tsp. prepared horseradish

Instructions:

1. In a small bowl, combine horseradish and mayonnaise and stir well.
2. Put some mayonnaise mixture on the bread.
3. Arrange the roast beef slices and spinach on a bread slice and top it with the other bread.
4. Serve the sandwich with slices of cucumber with dressing.

Kale Fried Rice

Ingredients:

- 2 tbsp. coconut oil
- 2 whole eggs
- 2 large garlic cloves, minced
- 3 large green onions, thinly sliced
- 1 cup of carrots, cut into matchsticks
- 1 cup of Brussels sprouts, diced
- 1 medium bunch of kale, ribs removed and the leaves shredded
- 2 cups brown rice, cooked and cooled
- 1/4 tsp. Himalayan salt
- 1/4 cup of lemon balm leaves, diced
- 3/4 cups of shredded coconut, unsweetened variety
- fresh cilantro, for garnishing

Instructions:

1. Heat up a teaspoon of oil in a large skillet over medium-high heat.
2. Pour in the egg mixture.
3. Cook the eggs while occasionally stirring.
4. Remove from the pan and set aside.
5. Pour another teaspoon of coconut oil into the pan, along with Brussels sprouts, carrots, garlic, and green onions.

6. Stir every now and then until the vegetables look tender.
7. Add kale and salt.
8. Remove from the pan and put them into where the egg is.
9. Put the remaining coconut oil into the pan. Add in coconut flakes, stirring frequently
10. Add rice and stir it in.
11. Add the egg and vegetable mixture to the pan, as well as the lemon balm leaves.
12. Stir to combine and heat through.
13. Transfer to a serving bowl and garnish with fresh cilantro.
14. Serve and enjoy.

Stir-Fried Cabbage and Apples

Ingredients:

- 1 shallot, thinly sliced
- 1/2 apple, cut into cubes
- 1/4 savoy cabbage, sliced thinly into strips
- 3–4 radishes, sliced thinly
- 1/2–1 tsp. coconut oil
- salt, to taste

Instructions:

1. Pour some coconut oil into a wok.
2. Add shallot and cook until translucent.
3. Add the cabbage, radish, and apples to the wok.
4. Stir-fry for about 5 minutes. Don't overcook.
5. Add salt to taste.
6. Serve while warm.

Roast Broccoli and Salmon

Ingredients:

- 1 bunch broccoli, cut into florets
- 4 tbsp. canola oil, divided
- salt
- pepper
- 4 pcs. salmon filets, skins removed
- 1 pc. jalapeño or red fresno chile, seeds removed, sliced into thin rings
- 2 tbsp. rice vinegar, unseasoned
- 2 tbsp. capers, drained

Instructions:

1. Preheat the oven to 400° F.
2. On a large, rimmed baking sheet, put the broccoli florets and toss in 2 tablespoons of the canola oil. Season with salt and pepper.
3. Roast the florets in the oven for 12 or 15 minutes. Toss occasionally.
4. Remove from the oven when the florets are crisp-tender and browned.
5. Gently rub the filets with 1 tablespoon of the canola oil. Season the salmon with salt and pepper.
6. Put the salmon in the middle of the baking sheet.

7. Move the florets to the sides of the baking sheet. Roast the filet for 10 to 15 minutes or until the filets turn opaque throughout.
8. In a small bowl, combine the vinegar, chile rings, and a pinch of salt.
9. Let the mixture sit for about 10 minutes so that the chile rings become somewhat softened,
10. Add the capers and the remaining tablespoon of canola oil. Add salt and pepper to taste.
11. Drizzle chile vinaigrette over the roasted broccoli and salmon just before serving.

Asian-Themed Macrobiotic Bowl

Ingredients:

- 2 cups cooked quinoa
- 4 carrots
- 1 package of smoked tofu
- 1 tbsp. nutritional yeast
- 2 tbsp. coconut aminos
- 4 tbsp. sunflower sprouts
- 2 tbsp. fermented vegetables
- 1 cup of shiitake mushrooms
- 1 avocado
- 2 tbsp. hemp seeds
- 2-3 cooked beets
- coconut oil cooking spray

Dressing:

- 2 tbsp. miso paste
- 1 tbsp. tahini
- 1 clove garlic, crushed
- 1 tbsp. olive oil
- 1/2 lime, juiced
- 3 tbsp. water

Instructions:

1. Roast the carrots in the oven at 400°F for 30-40 minutes.

2. Wash the vegetables, trim, and spray them with coconut oil.
3. Add them to the oven. When they are cooked, set them aside till you are ready to assemble the Buddha bowl.
4. Make the dressing by combining all of the ingredients in a medium-sized bowl. If the dressing appears lumpy, add more water.
5. To build the bowl, put the quinoa on the bottom and then arrange the vegetables on top.
6. Sprinkle the bowls with hemp seeds and drizzle the dressing over top.
7. Now serve and enjoy!

Spinach Quiche

Ingredients:

- 1 lb. breakfast sausage
- 1/2 onion, diced
- 2 cups mushrooms, sliced
- 6 cups spinach, roughly chopped
- 12 eggs
- 1/4 to 1/2 cup full-fat coconut milk
- 1 tsp. garlic powder
- 1 tsp. Italian seasoning
- 1 tsp. salt
- 1 tsp. pepper

Instructions:

1. Preheat the oven to 400°F.
2. Heat a cast-iron pan or another oven-safe pan over medium heat.
3. Cook sausage and onion. Stir occasionally until sausage turns brown, about 7-8 minutes.
4. Add in mushrooms. Allow them to cook with the sausage until soft, for about 2 minutes. Remove from heat.
5. Crack eggs into a large bowl.
6. Add coconut milk. For a lighter and fluffier texture, use ½ cup. Use less for less coconut taste.
7. Whisk together well to get a light egg mixture.

8. Add spinach and seasonings to the bowl with the eggs.
9. Add the sausage mixture to the bowl with the rest of the ingredients.
10. Mix until everything is well blended.
11. Line the pan with some fat from the sausage or grease well with oil, butter, or ghee to prevent the quiche from sticking.
12. Pour the mixture into the cast iron pan or oven-safe dish.
13. Bake for 40-45 minutes or until a knife poked at the center comes out clean.
14. Serve and enjoy while warm.

Grilled Eggplant

Ingredients:

- 2 small eggplants or 1 large eggplant, around 1-1/4 to 1-1/12 lb. in total, sliced into half-inch-thick rounds
- 2 tbsp. extra-virgin olive oil
- salt

Instructions:

1. Preheat the grill using the medium-high setting.
2. Toss eggplant slices and olive oil in a bowl.
3. Sprinkle it with salt to taste.
4. Toss ingredients again.
5. Place eggplant slices onto the grill.
6. Turn over to the other side after about 4 minutes, or until charred spots have appeared on the underside.
7. Continue grilling until eggplant slices have become tender.
8. When storing, place into an airtight container once it has cooled down, and then refrigerate. Grilled eggplant can last for up to 4 days in a chilled condition.

Conclusion

Acne keloidalis nuchae, also known as AKN, is a condition that manifests itself as raised bumps on the nape of the neck. AKN is frequently brought on by constricted hairstyles, frequent shaving, and long, hot showers.

There is currently no treatment that can reverse the effects of AKN, but there are ways to manage the condition and cut down on its symptoms. The bumps on the skin can be reduced and the overall appearance of the skin can be improved with the help of a healthy diet and natural treatments.

In addition, if you want to lessen the severity of the symptoms of AKN, you should avoid getting your hair cut too short, shaving, and taking very hot showers. Discuss the various treatment options with your physician if you are having trouble keeping your AKN under control.

FAQ About Acne Keloidalis Nuchae

What causes AKN?

The exact cause of AKN is unknown, but it is often associated with tight hairstyles, shaving, and hot showers.

Is there a cure for AKN?

There is no cure for AKN, but there are ways to manage the condition and reduce the symptoms.

How can I reduce the bumps associated with AKN?

A healthy diet and natural treatments can help to reduce the bumps and improve the appearance of the skin. In addition, avoiding tight hairstyles, shaving, and hot showers can help to reduce the symptoms of AKN.

I am struggling to manage my AKN. What should I do?

If you are struggling to manage your AKN, talk to your doctor about treatment options. Several natural treatments can help to reduce the bumps and improve the appearance of the skin. In addition, several lifestyle changes can help to reduce the symptoms of AKN. These lifestyle changes include avoiding tight hairstyles, shaving, wearing loose clothing, and avoiding hot showers.

References and Helpful Links

Acne keloidalis nuchae: What it is, causes & treatment. (n.d.). Retrieved August 12, 2022, from https://my.clevelandclinic.org/health/diseases/22891-acne-keloidalis-nuchae.

Acne keloidalis—Scalp bump—Scars—Black skin care. (n.d.). Retrieved August 12, 2022, from https://clinicallyclear.com/acne-keloidalis.

Kukreja, K. (2019, July 4). What is acne keloidalis nuchae and how to treat it? https://www.olivaclinic.com/blog/acne-keloidalis-nuchae-causes-treatments-in-india/.

Maranda, E. L., Simmons, B. J., Nguyen, A. H., Lim, V. M., & Keri, J. E. (2016). Treatment of acne keloidalis nuchae: A systematic review of the literature. Dermatology and Therapy, 6(3), 363–378. https://doi.org/10.1007/s13555-016-0134-5.

Managing acne keloidalis nuchae (Akn). (n.d.). Retrieved August 12, 2022, from https://www.britishskinfoundation.org.uk/blog/managing-acne-keloidalis-nuchae-akn.

www.ingramcontent.com/pod-product-compliance
Lightning Source LLC
LaVergne TN
LVHW051925060526
838201LV00062B/4683